The
Essential Walker's
Journal

The Essential Walker's Journal

Your Companion to Weight Loss, Health, and Personal Transformation

Leslie Sansone
with Rowan Jacobsen

CENTER
STREET

New York   Boston   Nashville

Copyright © 2006 by Walk Aerobics, Inc.

Center Street

Time Warner Book Group
1271 Avenue of the Americas, New York, NY 10020
Visit our website at www.twbookmark.com

The Center Street name and logo are registered trademarks of the Time Warner Book Group.

Printed in the United States of America

First edition: April 2006

10 9 8 7 6 5 4 3 2 1

ISBN: 0-446-69336-7
Library of Congress Control Number: 2005932217

CONTENTS

I'VE GOT GREAT NEWS FOR YOU! The simple fact that you have bought this journal means you are very likely to succeed. Studies show that the *very best indicator* that people will reach their fitness goals is the use of an exercise journal. People who use fitness journals are much more likely to create a plan and stay focused on it. A little attention each day is what makes the difference.

I created this journal after hearing from women who loved the structured exercise goals they found in my first book and the structured eating plan they found in my second, and wanted a way of maintaining that structure as they continued to walk away from excess weight and toward a life of health and happiness. If you're like me, structure is your key to staying on task, no matter what the project. That's because with structure comes the ability to stick to goals, to see your progress, to stay motivated, and to recognize patterns you might not realize you had. Maybe you're the type who does much better exercising in the evening. Maybe you feel better after two-mile walks than you do after three-mile walks. Maybe that afternoon coffee is affecting your sleep. Logging a few weeks in this journal can help to make all those patterns clear.

Many women who participate in my Walk Diets are amazed how at the end of a few weeks they are walking three miles with ease, while back at Week 1, they struggled to complete a mile. That's the kind of pleasure I want you to get from this journal. When you can flip through the pages and see how much you improve week to week, it makes all the difference in motivating you to continue.

That said, I want this journal to be about much more than just tracking your daily exercise. Exercise does not happen in a vacuum; it happens when you make the time in your daily life to do it, and it can't be separated from all the other things that make up your daily life. Eating, sleeping, and maintaining a positive outlook are all vital aspects of maintaining a healthy lifestyle—which is our ultimate reason for exercising, isn't it? I want this journal to be your companion to a life of healthy living, to be a single place you can go to, not only to record your workouts, meals, and thoughts, but also to plan your future and make sure you keep getting closer to that vision of the ideal healthy person you want to be.

Here's another interesting tidbit from the researchers: Writing down your feelings actually boosts your immunity to illness and reduces muscle pain, headaches, and fatigue. Of course, those of us who are lifelong diary keepers probably suspected that all along. If you aren't a diary writer, try jotting down a few thoughts and feelings in this journal. You may be amazed at how it lightens your load.

The other reason I like to write down feelings is because exploring our feelings helps us get a handle on who we are and what we really want out of life. This book is all about turning your dreams into reality. We all have hopes and aspirations that float through our minds during the busy day but are gone by evening, replaced by thoughts about what to cook for dinner and where the car keys could possibly be. Catching those little seeds as they float by and planting them in the rich dreaming ground of a journal is the first step toward bringing them out of the realm of could-be and letting them flower.

Use this journal as your garden of hopes. Let it help you to cultivate them and to grow your dream. The more you put into it, the lusher that dream will get, and the closer you will get to it. By the time you have filled all the pages in this book, you may look around and realize that you are living your dream every day.

The
Essential Walker's
Journal

How to Use This Journal

THE MOST IMPORTANT THING TO KNOW about using this journal is to *relax*. This is *your* journal, to be used however you see fit. Nobody is going to check your answers or make sure you filled in every page, because there is no one way of keeping a journal that works for everybody. Some people like journals with completely blank pages. Others want slots in which to write in their key numbers—miles, heart rate, whatever—and aren't comfortable with free space at all. I've tried to strike a balance here so that you can customize the pages to suit your needs. Each day has places to record all the things you do if you follow my program: your walking, strength training, water consumption, multivitamin, and sleep. It also has space to keep track of your eating if you choose to do so.

Each page includes some free space to use as you see fit: Explore your moods, get out your frustrations, or write down a list of the healthy whole foods you need to pick up at the store tomorrow.

BEFORE YOU BEGIN: VERBALIZE YOUR GOALS

The first step in realizing your dreams is nailing down what those dreams are and charting a course to get there. That is where the Dreamweaver page comes in. It's your chance to indulge yourself and go for broke. Write down what you *really* want to weigh, look like, feel like, and be able to do in life. You can't start on a journey unless you have a direction to go in; this is where you set up a star to guide you.

RECORD YOUR VITAL STATS

I have mixed feelings about numbers. They can never express how someone really looks and feels, and they can be misleading. The same weight can look very different on different people, depending on height, bone structure, and even ratio of fat to muscle, because muscle weighs more than fat. Still, numbers are the best way we have of tracking progress. If your cholesterol level has dropped twenty points after a month of exercising and eating right, you *know* you've been doing good work. I like people to start off this journal by recording whatever numbers are most important for their personal health, whether it's weight, blood pressure, or glucose level. Then, each month, I ask them to check in and see how much progress they've made.

READ THE NUTSHELLS

The sections in the chapter entitled "The Nutshells" provide basic information on weight loss, nutrition, and fitness. It's good to know why you're doing what you're doing! If you want to know more, you can find complete explanations and instructions for every aspect of working out, staying healthy, eating right, and staying motivated in my books *Walk Away the Pounds* and *Eat Smart, Walk Strong*.

THE DAY PAGES

These are similar to the Day Pages from my six-week weight-loss programs. They can fulfill a variety of needs. You can track your eating as well as your exercise, and you can use the journal to explore your feelings and goals, or even just to keep track of daily events. Here's a rundown of what you'll find on those pages:

Thought for the Day

I love starting off my day by reading something wise, inspiring, or heartfelt. If I can begin my morning that way, it helps set the tone for the whole day. You're less likely to veer off into negative thoughts or general grumpiness. Each day in the journal starts off with some words to get you started. Sometimes I'll quote somebody else's wonderful Words to Live By; sometimes it will be a fascinating Fit Fact to remind you of the great benefits of exercise; sometimes it will feature the nutritional benefits of a Fab Food you might want to work into your diet; and other times I'll ask a question to trigger some Reflection as you go about your day. Whatever the words for that day, try reading them as soon as you wake up and see if that helps get you going even *before* you've had your coffee!

Today's Walk

This is where you record your miles walked, any upper-body strength training you did, your stretching before and after walking, and your general success. You can track the distance you walk, the time, or the steps you take (using a pedometer). Just remember this formula:

1 mile = 20 moderate minutes = 15 brisk minutes = 2,000 steps.

Obviously, the goal is to keep increasing the amount of exercise you get, but if you are walking three miles five times a week or so, and are mixing in some upper-body work half the time, you are getting all the exercise you need to stay healthy and in shape. If you are walking that much and still not losing weight, your diet is probably to blame. See "Weight Loss in a Nutshell" (page 20) for more information.

For a complete guide to basic walking steps, stretching routines, and a variety of strength-training workouts, see *Walk Away the Pounds*. And don't forget that you should always check with your doctor before beginning a fitness program of any kind.

Multivitamin and Hours of Sleep

If you use a day planner at work, you know how good it feels to check off the tasks completed for that day. Seems silly, but it works. It's like a little pat on the back. I know, you could probably manage to take a multivitamin each day without a reminder in your fitness journal, but why miss the chance for an extra pat? And you *should* pat yourself on the back, because a multivitamin truly can improve your health. Even if we eat an excellent diet, it's difficult for us to get enough of vitamins B_6, B_{12}, D, E, and folate through our food. Pick any multivitamin that meets the RDA requirements and you are reducing your risk of cardiovascular disease for just a few cents a day.

Getting enough sleep is even more important to good health than taking a multivitamin, yet most of us don't get what we need. Sleep is the time when the body repairs itself, defuses stress, and makes sure all systems are running smoothly. When we don't get enough sleep, we get less done at work, drive worse, look worse, and feel depressed about it all. We also don't metabolize glucose efficiently, meaning that sleep deprivation can mimic diabetes and lead to weight gain and heart disease. Most of us need eight to nine hours of sleep a night but get fewer than seven. This journal is a great opportunity to pay more attention to your sleep habits and discover if some changes can help you realize the full appreciation of life, which can come only with a full night's rest.

A Beautiful Thing

People loved this so much in my first book that I wanted to include it here, too. It's a great tool for getting your mental outlook as fit as your body. Use this space to record something beautiful that you see each day. This can be anything at all, from a crab-apple tree in full bloom to the smile on your child's face when you make blueberry pancakes for breakfast. What you are really doing with this exercise is training your mind to see the beauty that is already there in everyday things. It gets easy to ignore that beauty if it gets buried under the daily drum of bad news in the papers and on TV, but don't ignore it. Good things happen all around you; allow yourself to appreciate them when they do.

Nutrition Center

Most people who start exercising regularly end up naturally wanting to eat better, too. Ultimately, the two issues are sides of the same weight-loss coin, and you need to control both for long-lasting health and weight control. (Experts estimate that lack of exercise is responsible for 50 percent of America's weight problem, while overeating accounts for an additional 30 percent.) My second book, *Eat Smart, Walk Strong,* tells you everything you need to know about eating right and gives you lots of tips for developing healthy habits that will help you to lose weight without dieting struggles.

If you have already completed one of my books or Walk Diets, you may already be tracking your eating habits. Each Day Page includes space for you to continue to record meals, snacks, and water consumption. See "Nutrition in a Nutshell" (page 25) if you need basic information on eating right.

Notes

Here is that free space I promised you. Use this any way you see fit. Write poetry or grocery lists. Ignore it if you like. Use it instead of the structured space if you find yourself craving some diary time.

Where's Sunday?

In our household, Sundays are different from the rest of the week. We take things a little slower, don't make too many plans, and give ourselves a chance to relax and reflect on where we are. That's what Sundays are for in my program, too. It's important when exercising to take regular days off. This gives your muscles a chance to recover and build themselves back up. Equally important, it gives your mind a break from routine, which is essential for keeping things feeling fresh.

Don't worry about exercising or paying attention to your diet on Sundays. Just relax and go where the day takes you. I feel so strongly about having this free day that I didn't even put Sunday pages in the journal. Ha! You'll have to relax.

Of course, it's possible that your schedule makes Sunday one of the best days of the week for you to exercise. If so, then by all means feel free to pick a different day of the week as your free day. Just make sure you do have one. Whatever day of the week you pick as your free day, use that day's pages in the journal to record your Sunday workout, eating, and so on.

MONTHLY CHECK-IN

Every four weeks it's a good idea to do the numbers. Weight, cholesterol, glucose—whatever numbers are your personal keys to health and fitness, you can record them monthly. At your Monthly Check-In, it also helps to make sure you're on schedule for achieving your goals and, if not, to reaffirm your action plan for meeting them. These pages give you the space to do that.

FOUR-MONTH WRAP-UP

When you reach the end of this journal, the differences in your physical and mental makeup will be too profound for a mere monthly check-in. To do them justice, please complete the Four-Month Wrap-Up at the end of the book to get a complete picture of where you're at, how far you've come, and where you're going next.

Walking Wonder

Kari Andonov
PHOENIX, ARIZONA

Lost 79 pounds

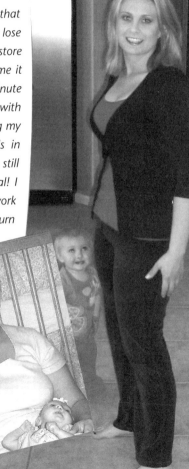

After the birth of my third child, I weighed in at 227 pounds. Being only five three, that was a huge load to carry. I woke up one day and it clicked in my head that I needed to do something; there was no reason for me to be that big. In the past, I had tried everything to lose weight and nothing worked. I went to the store and bought an exercise tape—lucky for me it was Leslie's! I started with one twenty-minute mile. Now I can do the four-mile walk with ease. By walking with Leslie and watching my calorie intake, I lost seventy-nine pounds in seven months! I now weigh 148 and am still on my quest. I know I will make my goal! I love to pop in one of Leslie's videos and work out with all the friendly, familiar faces. Burn more calories than you take in is the bottom line—and exercise is the key to help you to achieve that goal!

Dreamweaver

THE FIRST STEP IN ACHIEVING YOUR DREAMS is having some! So often, from the time we're children, we're encouraged to "get real," to stop dreaming and settle for whatever is within reach. I don't think that's healthy. The people who succeed wildly in life are the ones who dream big and then follow through with all the little things necessary to make their dreams come true. True, you have to have the commitment to do the little things, day in and day out—that's where this journal comes in! But you also need to have the dreams in the first place.

On the two Dreamweaver pages, please jot down all your hopes and aspirations for the person you wish to be in four months, a year, five years, whatever. Think big! If your goal is to lose twenty pounds of fat, write that down, but go further than that. Want to run a 5K race? To go hiking in the mountains with your kids? To appear in my next walking video? Write it all down.

Many of your goals will go beyond walking. Maybe you want to control your diabetes without using insulin. Maybe you want to get off your medication for high blood pressure. Maybe you just want to reduce stress so that you can be the best parent of all time. Those are all excellent goals! Perhaps you want to start your own company, and you know that to do it you'll need the energy and confidence that come from getting physically fit. Perhaps you dream about finding more spirituality in life and know that a healthy body is more receptive to spirit.

All right, I'll stop making suggestions now. These are *your* dreams, after all. My dream is that this journal will help you to find fulfillment by living a healthy, active, and meaningful life. And that's a dream I *know* can come true!

My Dreams
(Small, Medium, Big, and Downright Crazy)

or

Everything I Ever Dreamed about
but Was Afraid to Ask For

_____

_____

_____

_____

_____

_____

_____

_____

_____

_____

_____

_____

_____

_____

_____

_____

_____

_____

_____

My Vital Stats

YOU DON'T NEED TO FILL IN all of the numbers suggested here. Just record the ones most meaningful to your personal health. If your only goal is to lose ten pounds, weight might be all you care about. If you have diabetes, on the other hand, you'll want to record weight, glucose level, and probably blood pressure. Whatever numbers you choose to track, record those same numbers on the Monthly Check-In pages at the end of every four weeks, but come back *here* to fill in your final numbers after four months, because it's always such a kick to see those before and after numbers side by side and realize what progress you've made!

Most of us tend to focus on weight as the best measure of our improvement in fitness, but I think dress size may be a better yardstick. Muscle weighs more than fat, so as you lose fat and build muscle, you don't lose weight as quickly as you do *inches,* and since looking good (along with feeling good) is the goal, getting trim is more meaningful than some arbitrary number on a scale.

Before	After
Weight _____	Weight _____
Dress Size _____	Dress Size _____
Waist _____	Waist _____
Hips _____	Hips _____
Resting Heart Rate _____	Resting Heart Rate _____
Blood Pressure _____	Blood Pressure _____
Glucose _____	Glucose _____
Total Cholesterol _____	Total Cholesterol _____
LDL Cholesterol _____	LDL Cholesterol _____
Other _____	Other _____

The Nutshells

JOURNALS ARE FOR WRITING, not *reading,* and you may already be a weight-loss expert, but if you are at all hazy about the basic concepts behind weight loss, fitness, and nutrition, the following "nutshell" reports will quickly give you all the information you need to move forward confidently with your fitness goals.

WEIGHT LOSS IN A NUTSHELL

Don't believe a lot of the things you hear about weight loss. You don't need to go on some crazy no-carb diet to achieve it. You don't need to work yourself into a sweating lump of exhaustion every day, either. And you *definitely* don't need to take any dangerous diet pills. You just need to make some simple changes in lifestyle, and the weight will start to come off. This is true no matter how out of shape you are. In fact, the more overweight you are, the *faster* the weight will disappear. I know plenty of women who have lost one hundred pounds or more on my program, simply by walking and eating sensibly.

The key to weight loss is understanding the concept of energy balance. If calories consumed (through food) equal calories being burned (through metabolism and exercise), your weight will stay the same. If you consume more calories per day than you burn, your body stores the extra calories as fat. However, if you consume fewer calories per day than you burn, your body uses those fat stores to make up the difference. Presto! No more extra fat! That is our goal. This goal *can* be achieved through dieting alone, but almost nobody manages to. Here's why:

The Diet Dilemma

For most Americans, dieting is an essential part of weight loss because we consume many more calories per day than we can ever hope to burn off through exercise. That's because our meals have grown larger and less healthful than ever before. Supersized fast-food meals, all-you-can-eat buffets, and ultrasugary breakfast cereals all contribute to this problem. Constant snacking makes it much worse. Add in some high-calorie soft drinks and desserts every day, and you have the recipe for a daily caloric explosion that lands squarely on America's thighs and hips.

Most diets try to get you to lose weight by simply cutting back on your calorie intake. Eat less! This seems obvious—and most of us *do* need to consume fewer calories—but it's a bit more complicated than that. When you cut back on calories for a long time, you feel hungry all the time, and are likely to binge; and also, your body begins to think that food is scarce and goes into survival mode by lowering your metabolism until the "famine" is over. The result is that on most diets you lose some weight at first but then put it all back on later—and then some.

The Exercise Solution

Compare that scenario to what happens when you increase your daily exercise. Instead of being stored as fat, those food calories get burned by your muscles for energy. And because muscles constantly use energy (while fat doesn't), your metabolism goes up, so you burn more calories all the time, even when resting. You might think that this increased metabolism would mean you are always hungry, but it doesn't. Exercise regulates appetite. By burning sugars for fuel and by producing bigger muscles, exercise keeps your blood-sugar levels from rising fast, then dropping. A big drop in blood sugar is what causes hunger signals in the body.

So exercise is a win-win-win solution: You burn more calories and you tone muscle for a firmer, sleeker, younger look, yet you don't feel the need to eat more food, so you lose weight.

Of course, if you are eating three pints of ice cream a day (low-fat ice cream still has plenty of calories in it!), you are going to be hard-pressed to overcome that kind of calorie bomb through exercise. That's why most responsible programs, including mine, recommend a combination of controlled eating and daily exercise.

Slow and Steady

When you meet the real success stories—the people who lost a lot of weight and kept it off permanently—you notice they all have one thing in common: They didn't try to lose a ton of weight in two weeks. For example, they didn't fall for any miracle weight-loss pills. They committed themselves to lifestyle changes that resulted in a little bit of weight loss *every week*. That's where this journal comes in. I know it can help you to commit to a lifestyle of slow and steady progress that will lead to a new and wonderful you!

All You Need to Know

- The only way to lose weight is to burn more calories per day than you consume.
- It is easier to lose weight by increasing your daily exercise than by dieting.
- Dieting alone will never give you that firm, slender look you get through exercise.
- Exercise regulates blood-sugar levels, helping you to control your appetite.

FITNESS IN A NUTSHELL

I adore win-win situations, because they disprove that tired old notion that everything in life must be a trade-off. Notions like "Yummy food must be bad for you." Like "Getting fit and looking good involves a lot of sacrifice." Notions like "No pain, no gain."

That's not my style. My style is all gain, no pain. You

can eat delicious food that also gives your body all the nutrients it needs. And you can lead a lifestyle where fun and health are one and the same thing.

Take walking, for example. It's fun to do, and makes you feel really good when you're done. Not only does it help you to lose weight and look trim and beautiful; it also reduces your risk of virtually every major disease. The downside? In twenty-five years of walking, I've never found one!

People are often skeptical when they first hear of the amazing benefits of walking. They think, How could something so easy to do provide such impressive payback? It seems too good to be true, but the reasons why it is easy and why it is healthy are one and the same: because **we were designed to walk.** Our bodies are made to move, and we used to do it a lot before cars, sit-down lawn mowers, and remote controls took over for us.

What happens when you move frequently through regular exercise? You burn calories, of course, because your muscles use the food energy in your blood for fuel. To deliver the blood to your muscles, your heart pumps faster. If called on to do this regularly, your heart starts to get bigger and stronger so that it can pump more blood. Your muscles get bigger, too. And by frequently dilating to carry the extra blood, your blood vessels stay wide and flexible, meaning they are less likely to develop the cholesterol blockages that lead to strokes and heart disease.

Those are the most obvious benefits of exercise—greatly reduced risk of cardiovascular disease and diabetes, and increased metabolism—but there are also a host of secondary benefits, enough to fill a book.

- Exercise's mild pressure on your bones signals your body to make them bigger and stronger, helping to prevent osteoporosis.

- Excercise keeps your joints limber and arthritis-free.
- Exercise reduces stress that would otherwise leave you edgy.
- Exercise triggers endorphins in the brain that relieve mild depression.
- Exercise helps prevent asthma and Alzheimer's.
- Exercise boosts your immune system.

Great, you say, *but don't I need to run miles to get significant benefits?* Actually, walking is one of the healthiest exercises. Your body needs oxygen to turn fat supplies into fuel. Exercise that leaves you breathless doesn't burn fat, just sugar. Walking is perfect for keeping you at that optimum fat-burning pace where heart rate is up but you're not gasping. Mild, regular walking (thirty minutes a day, four days a week), plus some upper-body strength training for bone health, gives you all the benefits of exercise with virtually no risk of injury or exhaustion.

So don't think of exercise as a chore you do because it's good for you. Do what I do: Look forward to the great way it makes you feel and the extra energy it gives you, and just enjoy the health benefits as the flip side of the win-win situation that I call healthy living.

All You Need to Know

- Regular exercise dramatically reduces your risk of diabetes, heart disease, and stroke.
- Exercise helps to prevent depression, cancer, asthma, Alzheimer's disease, arthritis, and back pain.
- Moderate exercise such as walking provides the same health benefits as strenuous exercise.
- Strength training prevents osteoporosis and builds beautiful muscles.

Nutrition in a Nutshell

I grew up in a proud Italian-American family, and the very first lesson I learned about food has served me well my entire life: **Eating is a joyful part of living.** Food can be such an important part of family life. It can be a comfort and a pleasure and entertainment all rolled into one. Yet too often, food becomes a method of self-torture for us. We crave what we know we shouldn't have, or beat ourselves up for eating what we weren't supposed to.

To make matters worse, our brains are jammed every day with so many different messages on nutrition that it becomes impossible to know what we *should* be eating. Should it be low-fat food, low-carb food, or grapefruit at every meal? Should it be South Beach, Mediterranean, or L.A.? Eating becomes a loaded activity, filled with guilt and dread. And that is *not* a good plan.

I'm going to give you an excellent blueprint for a healthy life: *Eat, drink, and be merry!* To be more precise, eat lots of different good foods, drink lots of water, and approach life with a gracious, fun-filled attitude.

What constitutes "good food"? Probably a lot more things than you think. There are really only a handful of baddies to watch out for. Many of the things we thought we had to avoid ten years ago have turned out to be good for us. Here's a scorecard of some of the place switchers:

The Old Bad Guys	The New Bad Guys
Fats and Oils	Bread, Potatoes, Pasta,
Nuts	Cereal
Eggs	Dairy (full-fat)
Alcohol	

The Old Good Guys	The New Good Guys
Bread, Potatoes, Pasta, Cereal	Olive Oil
	Nuts
Dairy	Eggs
	Alcohol

What I like best about this list is that there are fewer bad guys and more good guys than there used to be. I love being able to enjoy the occasional omelette or glass of wine, and know I'm putting good nutrients in my body. And I love knowing that sensible eating is pretty much a matter of following common sense. As a general rule, you should consume plenty of fruits, veggies, whole grains (such as brown rice and whole-wheat bread), lean meat and fish, vegetable oils, nuts, and beans. Go easy on dairy, red meat, refined grains (white rice, white bread, and pasta), and sweets. Steer clear of transfats (anything with hydrogenated or partially hydrogenated oil in it) and pre-packaged foods as much as possible. Not so different from what our mothers told us when we were growing up!

The other essential part of the picture is portion control. I believe that most people's weight gain comes not so much from eating the wrong foods but from eating too much food, period. We all need to understand what a serving really is. A serving of meat, fish, or poultry should be around three ounces—about the size of a deck of cards. That T-bone drooping over the sides of the grill is a single serving—for the whole family! Keep yourself to the "one and done" rule—one plateful of food, no seconds—and you'll achieve weight control without even thinking about it. Once we get the idea out of our heads that we should rush back for seconds as soon as we've cleared our plates, we often find that we didn't really want those seconds after all. (If we can get rid of the idea that we need to clear our plates in the first place, even better.) My book *Eat Smart, Walk Strong* gives you lots of tricks to help get you started on a lifetime of portion control and smart eating.

All You Need to Know

- Exercise and portion control are the basis for maintaining a healthy weight.
- We feel hungry an hour or two after eating simple carbs (potatoes, white bread, white rice, pasta, and sweets) and then crave more of them, which is why these foods are the number-one cause of weight gain.
- Eating vegetables and whole grains at almost every meal, and making fruit your dessert of choice, will keep you on the right track.
- Cutting high-calorie drinks (sodas, juices, sweetened tea or coffee, and beer) and desserts from your diet is the easiest way to reduce your daily calories dramatically.

Walking Wonder

Barb Evans

PITTSBURGH, PENNSYLVANIA

Lost 130 pounds

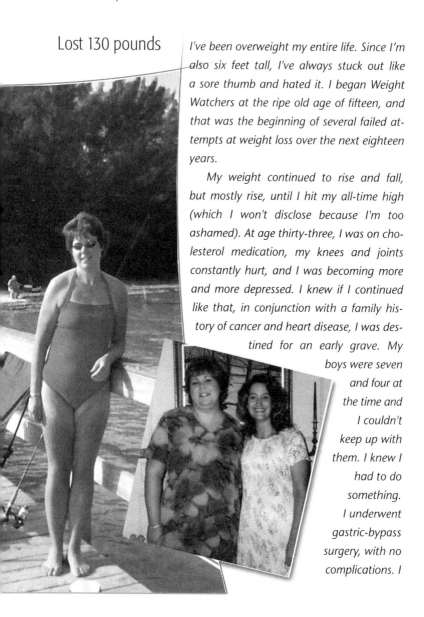

I've been overweight my entire life. Since I'm also six feet tall, I've always stuck out like a sore thumb and hated it. I began Weight Watchers at the ripe old age of fifteen, and that was the beginning of several failed attempts at weight loss over the next eighteen years.

My weight continued to rise and fall, but mostly rise, until I hit my all-time high (which I won't disclose because I'm too ashamed). At age thirty-three, I was on cholesterol medication, my knees and joints constantly hurt, and I was becoming more and more depressed. I knew if I continued like that, in conjunction with a family history of cancer and heart disease, I was destined for an early grave. My boys were seven and four at the time and I couldn't keep up with them. I knew I had to do something. I underwent gastric-bypass surgery, with no complications. I *knew the surgery itself was only a tool; my sedentary lifestyle had to change significantly if I wanted to be successful. Within four days of my surgery, I began taking short walks. Each day, I walked a little farther. My doctor was amazed at my determination.*

Three months after my surgery, I went on vacation with my cousin, who had recently purchased Walk Away the Pounds. *I gave it a try and LOVED IT! I began using the three-mile video five days a week while watching the weight melt from my body. At my six-month checkup, my surgeon couldn't believe how toned I was. Soon thereafter, I purchased the four-mile video and alternated it with the three-mile six to seven days a week. Today, almost two years later, I'm down 130 pounds. This is the longest I have ever persevered with an exercise program. I can honestly say I'm addicted.*

The weight-loss surgery got me on the right track, but walking with Leslie and maintaining healthy eating habits kept me on that track. I thank Leslie for her encouraging words and her simple exercises. I tell all my friends about her, and those who have tried her have had great success, as well. If I can do it, anyone can do it! I feel younger, happier, and much healthier than ever in my life. What I love most is that I can participate in my kids' activities and keep up!

The Day Pages

Words to Live By *"There is a woman at the beginning of all great things."* —ALPHONSE DE LAMARTINE, FRENCH POET

Today's Walk

How Far?_____

Strength Training? _____

How'd It Go?_____

Multivitamin ☐   Hours of Sleep ___

A Beautiful Thing

_____

_____

_____

Nutrition Center

Breakfast   Lunch

Dinner   Snacks

Drinks   Dessert

Water Log

① ② ③ ④ ⑤ ⑥ ⑦ ⑧

Notes _____

_____

_____

_____

Fit Fact — *The size and shape of your dishes can really affect how much you eat. Researchers find that people drink more from short, wide glasses than from tall, skinny ones, even though they think the tall glasses hold more. And people eat 50 percent more popcorn from large buckets than from smaller ones. Even if the popcorn is a day old! Use small bowls, plates, and glasses, and half your family's weight dilemma will be solved.*

Today's Walk

How Far?_____

Strength Training? _____

How'd It Go? _____

Multivitamin ☐   Hours of Sleep ____

A Beautiful Thing

_____

_____

_____

Nutrition Center

Breakfast   Lunch

Dinner   Snacks

Drinks   Dessert

Water Log

1   2   3   4   5   6   7   8

Notes _____

_____

Words to Live By *"The biggest change I've made is a spiritual one. It comes from the realization that taking care of my body and my health is really one of the greatest kinds of love I can give myself. Every day I put forth the effort to take care of myself. And there's no question I'm living a better life."* —OPRAH WINFREY, AMERICAN TV HOST

Today's Walk

How Far?_____

Strength Training? _____

How'd It Go? _____

Multivitamin ☐   Hours of Sleep ___

A Beautiful Thing

_____
_____
_____

Nutrition Center	
Breakfast	Lunch
Dinner	Snacks
Drinks	Dessert

Water Log

① ② ③ ④ ⑤ ⑥ ⑦ ⑧

Notes _____
_____

Fab Food — Red Cabbage

- *Excellent source of fiber and vitamin C*
- *High in indoles (phytonutrients that help to prevent breast cancer) and lycopene (phytonutrient that helps to prevent prostate cancer)*
- *Good source of beta-carotene, folate, and calcium*
- *A natural anti-inflammatory*
- *My favorite way to eat it: cole slaw*

Today's Walk

How Far?_____

Strength Training? _____

How'd It Go?_____

Multivitamin ☐   Hours of Sleep ____

A Beautiful Thing

_____
_____
_____

Nutrition Center	
Breakfast	Lunch
Dinner	Snacks
Drinks	Dessert

Water Log

1   2   3   4   5   6   7   8

Notes _____
_____

Words to Live By *"I am always doing things I can't do; that's how I get to do them."* —PABLO PICASSO, SPANISH ARTIST

Today's Walk

How Far?_____

Strength Training? _____

How'd It Go? _____

Multivitamin ☐　　　Hours of Sleep ___

A Beautiful Thing

_____

_____

_____

Nutrition Center

Breakfast　　　　　　Lunch

Dinner　　　　　　Snacks

Drinks　　　　　　Dessert

Water Log

1　2　3　4　5　6　7　8

Notes _____

_____

_____

_____

Reflections — *Did you grow up exercising and playing sports, or did you avoid them? Did you ever get a chance to enjoy them in a fun, noncompetitive environment? Think about what your relationship toward physical activity has been in your life, and what you can do to develop and improve that relationship.*

Today's Walk

How Far?_____

Strength Training? _____

How'd It Go?_____

Multivitamin ☐   Hours of Sleep ____

A Beautiful Thing

_____
_____
_____

Nutrition Center	
Breakfast	Lunch
Dinner	Snacks
Drinks	Dessert

Water Log

① ② ③ ④ ⑤ ⑥ ⑦ ⑧

Notes _____
_____
_____
_____

Words to Live By *"Everywhere is walking distance if you have the time."* —STEVEN WRIGHT, AMERICAN COMEDIAN

Today's Walk

How Far?_____

Strength Training? _____

How'd It Go? _____

Multivitamin ☐   Hours of Sleep ___

A Beautiful Thing

_____
_____
_____

Nutrition Center

Breakfast   Lunch

Dinner   Snacks

Drinks   Dessert

Water Log

1 2 3 4 5 6 7 8

Notes _____
_____
_____
_____

Fit Fact — The average woman today consumes 335 more calories per day than the average woman did thirty years ago. That works out to more than thirty pounds a year of extra weight!

Today's Walk

How Far?_____

Strength Training? _____

How'd It Go? _____

Multivitamin ☐   Hours of Sleep ____

A Beautiful Thing

_____
_____
_____

Nutrition Center

Breakfast	Lunch
Dinner	Snacks
Drinks	Dessert

Water Log

Notes _____
_____
_____
_____

Words to Live By *"It is no use walking anywhere to preach unless our walking is our preaching."*
—SAINT FRANCIS OF ASSISI, ITALIAN FRIAR

Today's Walk

How Far?_____

Strength Training? _____

How'd It Go? _____

Multivitamin ☐   Hours of Sleep ___

A Beautiful Thing

_____
_____
_____

Nutrition Center

Breakfast	Lunch
Dinner	Snacks
Drinks	Dessert

Water Log

1 2 3 4 5 6 7 8

Notes _____
_____
_____
_____
_____

Fab Food — Grapefruit

- *Excellent source of fiber, vitamin C, and flavonoids*
- *Good source of folate, potassium, lycopene, and beta-carotene*
- *May help prevent cancer and arthritis*
- *My favorite way to eat it: first thing in the morning*

Today's Walk

How Far?_____

Strength Training? _____

How'd It Go? _____

Multivitamin ☐   Hours of Sleep ___

A Beautiful Thing

_____

_____

_____

Nutrition Center

Breakfast	Lunch
Dinner	Snacks
Drinks	Dessert

Water Log

1 2 3 4 5 6 7 8

Notes _____

_____

_____

Words to Live By *"People often say that motivation doesn't last. Well, neither does bathing—that's why we recommend it daily."* —ZIG ZIGLAR, AMERICAN MOTIVATIONAL SPEAKER

Today's Walk

How Far?_____

Strength Training? _____

How'd It Go? _____

Multivitamin ☐   Hours of Sleep ___

A Beautiful Thing

_____

_____

_____

Nutrition Center	
Breakfast	Lunch
Dinner	Snacks
Drinks	Dessert

Water Log

1   2   3   4   5   6   7   8

Notes _____

_____

_____

_____

_____

Reflections — *Think about the people in the world you most admire. Write down their names in today's Notes section, then look over the list. What qualities do they have in common? Do you have those same qualities? What can you do to nurture them in yourself?*

Today's Walk

How Far?_____

Strength Training? _____

How'd It Go? _____

Multivitamin ☐   Hours of Sleep ____

A Beautiful Thing

_____

_____

_____

Nutrition Center

Breakfast	Lunch
Dinner	Snacks
Drinks	Dessert

Water Log

1   2   3   4   5   6   7   8

Notes _____

_____

_____

_____

Words to Live By *"Take care of your body with steadfast fidelity. The soul must see through these eyes alone, and if they are dim, the whole world is clouded."*
—JOHANN WOLFGANG VON GOETHE, GERMAN POET

Today's Walk

How Far?_____

Strength Training? _____

How'd It Go?_____

Multivitamin ☐   Hours of Sleep ___

A Beautiful Thing

_____
_____
_____

Nutrition Center	
Breakfast	Lunch
Dinner	Snacks
Drinks	Dessert

Water Log

Notes _____
_____
_____
_____

Fit Fact — *How much exercise do our modern conveniences cost us? To find out, researchers put pedometers on Amish farmers—who don't use cars, tractors, or phones. The results were eye-opening: The men averaged 18,000 steps per day, the women, 14,000. That's three times what most of us get! I'm not suggesting you give up your car entirely, but . . . maybe every now and then!*

Today's Walk

How Far?_____

Strength Training? _____

How'd It Go? _____

　　　Multivitamin ☐　　　Hours of Sleep ____

A Beautiful Thing

_____
_____
_____

Nutrition Center

Breakfast　　　　　　　Lunch

Dinner　　　　　　　　Snacks

Drinks　　　　　　　　Dessert

Water Log

1　2　3　4　5　6　7　8

Notes _____
_____
_____

Words to Live By *"Faith moves mountains, but you have to keeep pushing while you are praying."*

—MASON COOLEY, AMERICAN APHORIST

Today's Walk

How Far?_____

Strength Training? _____

How'd It Go? _____

Multivitamin ☐   Hours of Sleep ___

A Beautiful Thing

_____
_____
_____

Nutrition Center	
Breakfast	Lunch
Dinner	Snacks
Drinks	Dessert

Water Log

① ② ③ ④ ⑤ ⑥ ⑦ ⑧

Notes _____
_____
_____
_____
_____

Fab Food — Olive Oil

- *Excellent source of healthy, unsaturated fat*
- *Reduces cholesterol and helps to prevent heart disease*
- *Use sparingly: rich in calories*
- *My favorite way to eat it: drizzled over fresh greens with a little balsamic vinegar*

Today's Walk

How Far?_____

Strength Training? _____

How'd It Go? _____

     Multivitamin ☐   Hours of Sleep ___

A Beautiful Thing

_____

_____

_____

Nutrition Center	
Breakfast	Lunch
Dinner	Snacks
Drinks	Dessert

Water Log

Notes _____

_____

Words to Live By *"Striving for excellence motivates you; striving for perfection is demoralizing."*
—HARRIET BRAIKER, AMERICAN PSYCHOLOGIST

Today's Walk

How Far?_____

Strength Training? _____

How'd It Go? _____

Multivitamin ☐   Hours of Sleep ___

A Beautiful Thing

_____
_____
_____

Nutrition Center

Breakfast   Lunch

Dinner   Snacks

Drinks   Dessert

Water Log

1 2 3 4 5 6 7 8

Notes _____
_____
_____
_____
_____

Reflections — *Who are the people who play a role in supporting your physical, mental, and emotional health? Do you, in turn, support theirs? What can you do to acknowledge and honor that mutual support?*

Today's Walk

How Far?_____

Strength Training? _____

How'd It Go? _____

Multivitamin ☐   Hours of Sleep ____

A Beautiful Thing

_____
_____
_____

Nutrition Center

Breakfast	Lunch
Dinner	Snacks
Drinks	Dessert

Water Log

Notes _____
_____
_____
_____
_____

Words to Live By *"Never hurry. Take plenty of exercise. Always be cheerful. Take all the sleep you need. You may expect to be well."* —JAMES FREEMAN CLARKE, AMERICAN MINISTER

Today's Walk

How Far?_____

Strength Training? _____

How'd It Go? _____

Multivitamin ☐   Hours of Sleep ___

A Beautiful Thing

_____
_____
_____

Nutrition Center

Breakfast	Lunch
Dinner	Snacks
Drinks	Dessert

Water Log

1 2 3 4 5 6 7 8

Notes _____
_____
_____
_____

Fit Fact — *Those who walk every day have about half the risk of death from all causes compared to those who don't exercise.*

Today's Walk

How Far?_____

Strength Training? _____

How'd It Go? _____

Multivitamin ☐   Hours of Sleep ____

A Beautiful Thing

_____
_____
_____

Nutrition Center	
Breakfast	Lunch
Dinner	Snacks
Drinks	Dessert

Water Log

① ② ③ ④ ⑤ ⑥ ⑦ ⑧

Notes _____
_____
_____
_____
_____

Words to Live By *"I don't eat junk foods and I don't think junk thoughts."* —PEACE PILGRIM, AMERICAN PEACE ACTIVIST

Today's Walk

How Far?_____

Strength Training? _____

How'd It Go? _____

Multivitamin ☐   Hours of Sleep ___

A Beautiful Thing

_____

_____

_____

Nutrition Center

Breakfast	Lunch
Dinner	Snacks
Drinks	Dessert

Water Log

Notes _____

_____

_____

_____

_____

Fab Food — Mangoes

- Excellent source of vitamins A and C and fiber
- Good source of vitamin E, potassium, iron, and niacin
- My favorite way to eat them: dripping down my chin!

Today's Walk

How Far?_____

Strength Training? _____

How'd It Go?_____

Multivitamin ☐   Hours of Sleep ____

A Beautiful Thing

_____
_____
_____

Nutrition Center

Breakfast   Lunch

Dinner   Snacks

Drinks   Dessert

Water Log

① ② ③ ④ ⑤ ⑥ ⑦ ⑧

Notes _____
_____
_____
_____

Words to Live By *"The best way to know God is to love many things."* —VINCENT VAN GOGH, DUTCH PAINTER

Today's Walk

How Far?_____

Strength Training? _____

How'd It Go? _____

Multivitamin ☐   Hours of Sleep ____

A Beautiful Thing

_____
_____
_____

Nutrition Center

Breakfast   Lunch

Dinner   Snacks

Drinks   Dessert

Water Log

① ② ③ ④ ⑤ ⑥ ⑦ ⑧

Notes _____
_____
_____
_____
_____

Reflections — *Keeping a "gratitude journal" can be one of the most rewarding ways to remind ourselves of all the blessed things in life we usually take for granted. And being mindful of those things makes life all the sweeter. Use today's Notes section to make a list of five things you are grateful for.*

Today's Walk

How Far?_____

Strength Training? _____

How'd It Go? _____

Multivitamin ☐   Hours of Sleep ____

A Beautiful Thing

_____
_____
_____

Nutrition Center

Breakfast   Lunch

Dinner   Snacks

Drinks   Dessert

Water Log

1 2 3 4 5 6 7 8

Notes _____
_____
_____
_____

Monthly Check-In

Record below whichever numbers you've chosen to track, and compare with your original vital stats to see the improvement in your body in just one month. Then use the space provided to take stock of all that you have achieved. Note what you still need to work on—along with the *actions* you will take in the next month to realize those goals.

Weight	_____	**Dress Size**	_____
Waist	_____	**Hips**	_____
Resting Heart Rate	_____	**Blood Pressure**	_____
Glucose	_____	**Total Cholesterol**	_____
LDL Cholesterol	_____	**Other**	_____

Goals met or exceeded

_____

_____

_____

_____

_____

_____

_____

_____

_____

Goals that still need attention, and actions you will take to meet them

_____

_____

_____

_____

_____

_____

_____

_____

New goals or dreams

_____

_____

_____

_____

_____

_____

_____

_____

Walking Wonder

Bridget Sensabaugh

WILMINGTON, DELAWARE

I lost both of my parents in my early adult life because they didn't take good care of themselves. I was heading down the same road: I was having trouble with my knees and occasional chest pains. I have three children, and I didn't want to leave them motherless. My doctor tested me for diabetes and told me I needed to get the weight off to improve my overall health. The day after my physical, I started Walk Away the Pounds. *The thing I loved was that I could do it! At 222 pounds, there were so many things I couldn't do. I started off by doing one mile. I kept that up for about two weeks, working out at least six days a week. Then I moved up to two miles, three miles, and finally four miles. Last year was a particularly stressful year for me, yet amazingly, I didn't gain any weight! I think the walking really helped release some of the stress. I try and do my tapes in the mornings. That allows for "me" time, and I don't have to take time away from my children. It is so nice that someone has made a program for everyone—all ages and all shapes!*

Lost 90 pounds

Words to Live By *"My grandmother started walking five miles a day when she was sixty. She's ninety-seven now, and we don't know where the h*** she is."*

—ELLEN DEGENERES, AMERICAN COMEDIAN

Today's Walk

How Far?_____

Strength Training? _____

How'd It Go? _____

Multivitamin ☐   Hours of Sleep ___

A Beautiful Thing

_____
_____
_____

Nutrition Center	
Breakfast	Lunch
Dinner	Snacks
Drinks	Dessert

Water Log

Notes _____
_____
_____
_____

Fit Fact — Researchers find that people eat more than twice as much of a food if it's within hand's reach than they do if it's across the room. Getting rid of your home's cookie jars, chip bags, and candy bowls can eliminate hundreds of daily calories from your diet—without any further effort on your part!

Today's Walk

How Far?_____

Strength Training? _____

How'd It Go? _____

Multivitamin ☐   Hours of Sleep ____

A Beautiful Thing

_____
_____
_____

Nutrition Center

Breakfast   Lunch

Dinner   Snacks

Drinks   Dessert

Water Log

① ② ③ ④ ⑤ ⑥ ⑦ ⑧

Notes _____
_____
_____
_____

Words to Live By *"Walking is the best possible exercise. Habituate yourself to walk very far."*

—THOMAS JEFFERSON, AMERICAN PRESIDENT

Today's Walk

How Far?_____

Strength Training? _____

How'd It Go?_____

Multivitamin ☐   Hours of Sleep ___

A Beautiful Thing

_____
_____
_____

Nutrition Center

Breakfast   Lunch

Dinner   Snacks

Drinks   Dessert

Water Log

1 2 3 4 5 6 7 8

Notes _____
_____
_____
_____
_____

Fab Food — Shellfish

- *Excellent source of protein, zinc, iron, and B vitamins*
- *Low in fat and delicious*
- *My favorite way to eat it: shrimp scampi*

Today's Walk

How Far?_____

Strength Training? _____

How'd It Go? _____

Multivitamin ☐   Hours of Sleep ____

A Beautiful Thing

_____

_____

_____

Nutrition Center

Breakfast	Lunch
Dinner	Snacks
Drinks	Dessert

Water Log

① ② ③ ④ ⑤ ⑥ ⑦ ⑧

Notes _____

_____

_____

_____

Words to Live By *"Most of our obstacles would melt away if, instead of cowering before them, we should make up our minds to walk boldly through them."*

—ORISON SWETT MARDEN, AMERICAN AUTHOR

Today's Walk

How Far?_____

Strength Training? _____

How'd It Go?_____

Multivitamin ☐   Hours of Sleep ____

A Beautiful Thing

_____
_____
_____

Nutrition Center

Breakfast   Lunch

Dinner   Snacks

Drinks   Dessert

Water Log

Notes _____
_____
_____
_____

Reflections — Think about ways that the modern world prevents most people from staying physically active. What changes can you make in your own lifestyle to circumvent this? Write down all the ideas you come up with in today's Notes section.

Today's Walk

How Far?_____

Strength Training? _____

How'd It Go?_____

Multivitamin ☐   Hours of Sleep ____

A Beautiful Thing

_____
_____
_____

Nutrition Center	
Breakfast	Lunch
Dinner	Snacks
Drinks	Dessert

Water Log

1 2 3 4 5 6 7 8

Notes _____
_____
_____
_____

Words to Live By *"Finish each day and be done with it. You have done what you could; some blunders and absurdities have crept in; forget them as soon as you can. Tomorrow is a new day; you shall begin it serenely and with too high a spirit to be encumbered with your old nonsense."* —RALPH WALDO EMERSON, AMERICAN ESSAYIST

Today's Walk

How Far?_____

Strength Training? _____

How'd It Go? _____

Multivitamin ☐　　Hours of Sleep ___

A Beautiful Thing

_____
_____
_____

Nutrition Center

Breakfast	Lunch
Dinner	Snacks
Drinks	Dessert

Water Log

Notes _____
_____

Fit Fact — *It's best to drink a cup of water before exercising and a cup after. The cup before ensures that you have the water you need to transport energy to your muscle cells and to sweat as much as needed to maintain an even temperature. The cup after makes sure you didn't sweat more than you drank. Don't worry about sports drinks–they are just another way to consume empty calories, and the electrolytes they include are a part of any healthy diet already.*

Today's Walk

How Far?_____

Strength Training? _____

How'd It Go? _____

Multivitamin ☐   Hours of Sleep ____

A Beautiful Thing

_____
_____
_____

Nutrition Center	
Breakfast	Lunch
Dinner	Snacks
Drinks	Dessert

Water Log

Notes _____
_____

Words to Live By *"People see God every day; they just don't recognize Him."*

—PEARL BAILEY, AMERICAN SINGER AND ACTRESS

Today's Walk

How Far?_____

Strength Training? _____

How'd It Go? _____

Multivitamin ☐   Hours of Sleep ___

A Beautiful Thing

_____
_____
_____

Nutrition Center

Breakfast   Lunch

Dinner   Snacks

Drinks   Dessert

Water Log

1   2   3   4   5   6   7   8

Notes _____
_____
_____
_____
_____

Fab Food — Chilies

- *Excellent source of vitamins A and C and flavonoids*
- *May help to prevent blood clotting, stroke, and heart disease*
- *My favorite way to eat them: in fresh salsa*

Today's Walk

How Far?_____

Strength Training? _____

How'd It Go? _____

Multivitamin ☐   Hours of Sleep ____

A Beautiful Thing

_____
_____
_____

Nutrition Center

Breakfast	Lunch
Dinner	Snacks
Drinks	Dessert

Water Log

1   2   3   4   5   6   7   8

Notes _____
_____
_____
_____

Words to Live By   "*Nothing lifts me out of a bad mood better than a hard workout on my treadmill. It never fails. Exercise is nothing short of a miracle.*"

—CHER, AMERICAN SINGER

Today's Walk

How Far?_____

Strength Training? _____

How'd It Go?_____

Multivitamin ☐   Hours of Sleep ___

A Beautiful Thing

_____
_____
_____

Nutrition Center	
Breakfast	Lunch
Dinner	Snacks
Drinks	Dessert

Water Log

1   2   3   4   5   6   7   8

Notes _____
_____
_____
_____

Reflections — *What role does food play in your life? Do you use it as a reward, or to help yourself feel good? If so, when in your life did these feelings start, and what can you now do to break free of them?*

Today's Walk

How Far?_____

Strength Training? _____

How'd It Go? _____

Multivitamin ☐   Hours of Sleep ____

A Beautiful Thing

_____
_____
_____

Nutrition Center

Breakfast	Lunch
Dinner	Snacks
Drinks	Dessert

Water Log

1 2 3 4 5 6 7 8

Notes _____
_____
_____
_____

Words to Live By *"As long as you know what it is you desire, then by simply affirming that it is yours—firmly and positively, with no ifs, buts, or maybes—over and over again, from the minute you arise in the morning until the time you go to sleep at night, and as many times during the day as your work or activities permit, you will be drawn to those people, places, and events that will bring your desires to you."* —SCOTT REED, AMERICAN AUTHOR

Today's Walk

How Far?_____

Strength Training? _____

How'd It Go?_____

Multivitamin ☐   Hours of Sleep ___

A Beautiful Thing

_____

_____

Nutrition Center

Breakfast	Lunch
Dinner	Snacks
Drinks	Dessert

Water Log

Notes _____

Fit Fact — Exercise is just as effective as antidepressants
in treating mild depression.

Today's Walk

How Far?_____

Strength Training? _____

How'd It Go?_____

Multivitamin ☐   Hours of Sleep ___

A Beautiful Thing

_____
_____
_____

Nutrition Center

Breakfast	Lunch
Dinner	Snacks
Drinks	Dessert

Water Log

1 2 3 4 5 6 7 8

Notes _____
_____
_____
_____
_____

Words to Live By *"To lengthen thy life, lessen thy meals."*
—BENJAMIN FRANKLIN, AMERICAN STATESMAN

Today's Walk

How Far?_____

Strength Training? _____

How'd It Go?_____

Multivitamin ☐   Hours of Sleep ___

A Beautiful Thing

_____
_____
_____

Nutrition Center

Breakfast   Lunch

Dinner   Snacks

Drinks   Dessert

Water Log

Notes _____
_____
_____
_____
_____

Fab Food — Avocados

- Excellent source of good fat, vitamin E, and fiber
- Good source of vitamin B_6 and potassium
- Help prevent heart disease and reduce insulin response
- My favorite way to eat them: in sandwiches and salads

Today's Walk

How Far?_____

Strength Training? _____

How'd It Go? _____

Multivitamin ☐   Hours of Sleep ____

A Beautiful Thing

_____
_____
_____

Nutrition Center

Breakfast   Lunch

Dinner   Snacks

Drinks   Dessert

Water Log

1   2   3   4   5   6   7   8

Notes _____
_____
_____

Words to Live By *"The human body is the best picture of the human soul."* —LUDWIG WITTGENSTEIN, AUSTRIAN PHILOSOPHER

Today's Walk

How Far?_____

Strength Training? _____

How'd It Go? _____

Multivitamin ☐   Hours of Sleep ___

A Beautiful Thing

_____
_____
_____

Nutrition Center

Breakfast	Lunch
Dinner	Snacks
Drinks	Dessert

Water Log

1 2 3 4 5 6 7 8

Notes _____
_____
_____
_____
_____

Reflections — What role does spirituality play in your life? Many people find that knowing the body is the house of the spirit makes taking care of that body both easier and more essential. How does your attitude toward your body and spirit affect your daily decisions?

Today's Walk

How Far?_____

Strength Training? _____

How'd It Go? _____

Multivitamin ☐   Hours of Sleep ____

A Beautiful Thing

_____
_____
_____

Nutrition Center

Breakfast   Lunch

Dinner   Snacks

Drinks   Dessert

Water Log

Notes _____
_____
_____
_____

Words to Live By *"Love is a force more formidable than any other. It is invisible, it cannot be seen or measured, yet it is powerful enough to transform you in a moment, and offer you more joy than any material possession could."*
—BARBARA DE ANGELIS, AMERICAN RELATIONSHIP EXPERT

Today's Walk

How Far?_____

Strength Training? _____

How'd It Go?_____

Multivitamin ☐   Hours of Sleep ___

A Beautiful Thing

_____
_____
_____

Nutrition Center

Breakfast   Lunch

Dinner   Snacks

Drinks   Dessert

Water Log

1 2 3 4 5 6 7 8

Notes _____
_____

Fit Fact — *Women who walk two to three miles, five days per week, take 50 percent fewer sick days than women who don't exercise.*

Today's Walk

How Far?_____

Strength Training? _____

How'd It Go?_____

Multivitamin ☐   Hours of Sleep ____

A Beautiful Thing

_____
_____
_____

Nutrition Center

Breakfast   Lunch

Dinner   Snacks

Drinks   Dessert

Water Log

Notes _____
_____
_____
_____
_____

Words to Live By *"Health is the greatest gift, contentment the greatest wealth, faithfulness the best relationship."* —BUDDHA

Today's Walk

How Far?_____

Strength Training? _____

How'd It Go? _____

Multivitamin ☐   Hours of Sleep ___

A Beautiful Thing

_____
_____
_____

Nutrition Center	
Breakfast	Lunch
Dinner	Snacks
Drinks	Dessert

Water Log

1 2 3 4 5 6 7 8

Notes _____
_____
_____
_____
_____

Fab Food — Beans

- Excellent source of fiber
- Good source of protein, B vitamins, iron, magnesium, and potassium
- My favorite way to eat them: in veggie enchiladas

Today's Walk

How Far?_____

Strength Training? _____

How'd It Go? _____

Multivitamin ☐   Hours of Sleep ____

A Beautiful Thing

_____

_____

_____

Nutrition Center

Breakfast	Lunch
Dinner	Snacks
Drinks	Dessert

Water Log

1   2   3   4   5   6   7   8

Notes _____

_____

_____

_____

Words to Live By *"We are underexercised as a nation. We look instead of play. We ride instead of walk. Our existence deprives us of the minimum of physical activity essential for healthy living."* —JOHN F. KENNEDY, AMERICAN PRESIDENT

Today's Walk

How Far?_____

Strength Training? _____

How'd It Go?_____

Multivitamin ☐   Hours of Sleep ___

A Beautiful Thing

_____
_____
_____

Nutrition Center

Breakfast	Lunch
Dinner	Snacks
Drinks	Dessert

Water Log

1 2 3 4 5 6 7 8

Notes _____
_____
_____
_____

Reflections — *What role does fear play in your life? How often do you hold back from doing something out of fear of failure, of criticism, or of ridicule? This stems from your ego saying, It is all about me. Try replacing this notion with the realization that it is all about divine love, and see if the fear disappears.*

Today's Walk

How Far?_____

Strength Training? _____

How'd It Go?_____

Multivitamin ☐   Hours of Sleep ____

A Beautiful Thing

_____
_____
_____

Nutrition Center	
Breakfast	Lunch
Dinner	Snacks
Drinks	Dessert

Water Log

🥛1 🥛2 🥛3 🥛4 🥛5 🥛6 🥛7 🥛8

Notes _____
_____
_____
_____

Monthly Check-In

Record below whichever numbers you've chosen to track, and compare with your original vital stats to see the improvement in your body in two months. Then use the space provided to take stock of all that you have achieved. Note what you still need to work on—along with the *actions* you will take in the next month to realize those goals.

Weight	____	**Dress Size**	____
Waist	____	**Hips**	____
Resting Heart Rate	____	**Blood Pressure**	____
Glucose	____	**Total Cholesterol**	____
LDL Cholesterol	____	**Other**	____

Goals met or exceeded

_____

_____

_____

_____

_____

_____

_____

_____

_____

Goals that still need attention, and actions you will take to meet them

_____

_____

_____

_____

_____

_____

_____

_____

New goals or dreams

_____

_____

_____

_____

_____

_____

_____

_____

Walking Wonder

Lyndel Walker
Hesston, Kansas

Lost 125 pounds

I started losing weight in January 2003 by cutting back on portions, focusing on fresh fruits and vegetables, increasing my physical activity, and using a lot of prayer. In summer, I rode a bike and swam a lot, but when it started cooling off, I worried about how I would keep up my activities. I did not really want to join a health club and spend extra time away from home. I work full-time and commute, so I would much rather be at home when I can. I discovered Leslie's program and began doing it. It has not only kept me in shape but actually improved my conditioning! I tell everyone that Leslie is my new best friend—I spend time with her every day. I have lost a total of 125 pounds now, and still have about 10 to go. I went from a size 3X to 12/14.

I spent a couple of weeks in France and was actually able to buy an outfit (they don't have size 3X clothes in France). The village where my daughter lives has a statue of Mary above it, made by the man who made the Statue of Liberty. Two years ago, I struggled up the mountain that it is located on, but I had no breath left for climbing up inside the statue. This visit, I strolled up the mountain and practically sprinted up the inside of the statue.

I am thrilled to be so active. My husband and I just bought kayaks for this summer. I would not have dreamed of even trying to get in one before. My goal is to go parasailing for my birthday in July. I couldn't imagine getting off the ground before! I got Leslie's book and have recommended it to all my friends. I thank God for this program and all that it has done to improve the quality of my life. I never dreamed I would be in such good shape again! I know that it has added wonderful years to my life, and I am looking forward to walking with Leslie's and God's help right into great-grandmotherhood!

Words to Live By   *"God is at home; it's we who have gone out for a walk."* —MEISTER ECKEHART, GERMAN MYSTIC

Today's Walk

How Far?_____

Strength Training? _____

How'd It Go? _____

Multivitamin ☐   Hours of Sleep ____

A Beautiful Thing

_____

_____

_____

Nutrition Center	
Breakfast	Lunch
Dinner	Snacks
Drinks	Dessert

Water Log

① ② ③ ④ ⑤ ⑥ ⑦ ⑧

Notes _____

_____

_____

_____

_____

Fit Fact — Postmenopausal women lose 2 percent of their bone mass per year–unless they exercise! The same women who did strength training twice a week gained bone mass and cut their risk of hip fracture in half.

Today's Walk

How Far?_____

Strength Training? _____

How'd It Go? _____

Multivitamin ☐   Hours of Sleep ____

A Beautiful Thing

_____
_____
_____

Nutrition Center

Breakfast	Lunch
Dinner	Snacks
Drinks	Dessert

Water Log

1   2   3   4   5   6   7   8

Notes _____
_____
_____
_____
_____

Words to Live By *"It's easy to have faith in yourself and have discipline when you're a winner, when you're number one. What you've got to have is faith and discipline when you're not yet a winner."* —VINCE LOMBARDI, AMERICAN FOOTBALL COACH

Today's Walk

How Far?_____

Strength Training? _____

How'd It Go?_____

Multivitamin ☐　　Hours of Sleep ___

A Beautiful Thing

_____
_____
_____

Nutrition Center

Breakfast	Lunch
Dinner	Snacks
Drinks	Dessert

Water Log

Notes _____
_____
_____
_____

Fab Food — Eggs

- *Excellent source of protein and vitamin B$_{12}$*
- *Do not affect most people's cholesterol levels*
- *My favorite way to eat them: scrambled for breakfast*

Today's Walk

How Far?_____

Strength Training? _____

How'd It Go? _____

Multivitamin ☐   Hours of Sleep ___

A Beautiful Thing

_____
_____
_____

Nutrition Center

Breakfast   Lunch

Dinner   Snacks

Drinks   Dessert

Water Log

1 2 3 4 5 6 7 8

Notes _____
_____
_____
_____

Words to Live By *"Call it a clan, call it a network, call it a tribe, call it a family: Whatever you call it, whoever you are, you need one."*
—JANE HOWARD, AMERICAN JOURNALIST

Today's Walk

How Far?_____

Strength Training? _____

How'd It Go? _____

Multivitamin ☐   Hours of Sleep ___

A Beautiful Thing

_____

_____

_____

Nutrition Center

Breakfast   Lunch

Dinner   Snacks

Drinks   Dessert

Water Log

1   2   3   4   5   6   7   8

Notes _____

_____

_____

_____

Reflections — *Think about your reasons for wanting to lose weight. At some deep level, many people believe that if they can become thin, then all their problems will vanish. Yet that is rarely the case. Are you putting any extra meaning into your weight or eating issues?*

Today's Walk

How Far?_____

Strength Training? _____

How'd It Go? _____

Multivitamin ☐   Hours of Sleep ___

A Beautiful Thing

_____
_____
_____

Nutrition Center

Breakfast	Lunch
Dinner	Snacks
Drinks	Dessert

Water Log

Notes _____
_____
_____
_____

Words to Live By *"The concept of total wellness recognizes that our every thought, word, and behavior affects our greater health and well-being. And we, in turn, are affected not only emotionally but also physically and spiritually."* —GREG ANDERSON, AMERICAN AUTHOR

Today's Walk

How Far?_____

Strength Training? _____

How'd It Go?_____

Multivitamin ☐   Hours of Sleep ___

A Beautiful Thing

_____
_____
_____

Nutrition Center

Breakfast	Lunch
Dinner	Snacks
Drinks	Dessert

Water Log

1 2 3 4 5 6 7 8

Notes _____
_____
_____

Fit Fact — *A daily walk of two miles reduces your risk of diabetes by almost 60 percent.*

Today's Walk

How Far?＿＿＿＿＿＿＿＿＿＿＿＿＿＿＿＿＿＿＿＿＿＿＿＿＿

Strength Training? ＿＿＿＿＿＿＿＿＿＿＿＿＿＿＿＿＿＿＿＿＿

How'd It Go? ＿＿＿＿＿＿＿＿＿＿＿＿＿＿＿＿＿＿＿＿＿＿＿＿

Multivitamin ☐　　　Hours of Sleep ＿＿

A Beautiful Thing

＿＿＿＿＿＿＿＿＿＿＿＿＿＿＿＿＿＿＿＿＿＿＿＿＿＿＿＿＿＿＿
＿＿＿＿＿＿＿＿＿＿＿＿＿＿＿＿＿＿＿＿＿＿＿＿＿＿＿＿＿＿＿
＿＿＿＿＿＿＿＿＿＿＿＿＿＿＿＿＿＿＿＿＿＿＿＿＿＿＿＿＿＿＿

Nutrition Center

Breakfast	Lunch
Dinner	Snacks
Drinks	Dessert

Water Log

1　2　3　4　5　6　7　8

Notes ＿＿＿＿＿＿＿＿＿＿＿＿＿＿＿＿＿＿＿＿＿＿＿＿＿＿
＿＿＿＿＿＿＿＿＿＿＿＿＿＿＿＿＿＿＿＿＿＿＿＿＿＿＿＿＿＿＿
＿＿＿＿＿＿＿＿＿＿＿＿＿＿＿＿＿＿＿＿＿＿＿＿＿＿＿＿＿＿＿
＿＿＿＿＿＿＿＿＿＿＿＿＿＿＿＿＿＿＿＿＿＿＿＿＿＿＿＿＿＿＿
＿＿＿＿＿＿＿＿＿＿＿＿＿＿＿＿＿＿＿＿＿＿＿＿＿＿＿＿＿＿＿

Words to Live By *"Motivation is what gets you started. Habit is what keeps you going."*

—JIM RYUN, AMERICAN RUNNER AND CONGRESSMAN

Today's Walk

How Far?_____

Strength Training? _____

How'd It Go? _____

Multivitamin ☐   Hours of Sleep ___

A Beautiful Thing

_____

_____

_____

Nutrition Center	
Breakfast	Lunch
Dinner	Snacks
Drinks	Dessert

Water Log

① ② ③ ④ ⑤ ⑥ ⑦ ⑧

Notes _____

_____

_____

_____

Fab Food — Dark Chocolate

- *Excellent source of flavonoids*
- *May help prevent heart disease and stroke*
- *Contains mood-lifting chemicals*
- *Use sparingly: rich in calories*
- *My favorite way to eat it: anytime, anywhere!*

Today's Walk

How Far?_____

Strength Training? _____

How'd It Go? _____

Multivitamin ☐   Hours of Sleep ____

A Beautiful Thing

_____
_____
_____

Nutrition Center	
Breakfast	Lunch
Dinner	Snacks
Drinks	Dessert

Water Log

🥛1 🥛2 🥛3 🥛4 🥛5 🥛6 🥛7 🥛8

Notes _____
_____

Words to Live By *"Not all of us have to possess earthshaking talent. Just common sense and love will do."*
—MYRTLE AUVIL, AMERICAN JOURNALIST

Today's Walk

How Far?_____

Strength Training? _____

How'd It Go? _____

Multivitamin ☐   Hours of Sleep ___

A Beautiful Thing

_____
_____
_____

Nutrition Center	
Breakfast	Lunch
Dinner	Snacks
Drinks	Dessert

Water Log

① ② ③ ④ ⑤ ⑥ ⑦ ⑧

Notes _____
_____
_____
_____
_____

Reflections — *Does your daily environment give you cues that reinforce your fitness goals, or does it throw obstacles in your way? Make a list of the simple changes you could make in lifestyle or habits that would make it easier for you to stay on your fitness path.*

Today's Walk

How Far?_____

Strength Training? _____

How'd It Go? _____

Multivitamin ☐　　　Hours of Sleep ____

A Beautiful Thing

_____
_____
_____

Nutrition Center	
Breakfast	Lunch
Dinner	Snacks
Drinks	Dessert

Water Log

Notes _____
_____
_____
_____

Words to Live By *"Just as a small fire is extinguished by the storm whereas a large fire is enhanced by it, likewise a weak faith is weakened by predicament and catastrophes whereas a strong faith is strengthened by them."*
—VIKTOR FRANKL, AUSTRIAN PSYCHIATRIST

Today's Walk

How Far?_____

Strength Training? _____

How'd It Go?_____

Multivitamin ☐   Hours of Sleep ___

A Beautiful Thing

_____
_____
_____

Nutrition Center	
Breakfast	Lunch
Dinner	Snacks
Drinks	Dessert

Water Log

① ② ③ ④ ⑤ ⑥ ⑦ ⑧

Notes _____
_____
_____

Fit Fact — *The average person spends three hours per day watching TV but only twenty minutes exercising. Balance those numbers and you'll never have to worry about weight again.*

Today's Walk

How Far?_____

Strength Training? _____

How'd It Go? _____

Multivitamin ☐   Hours of Sleep ___

A Beautiful Thing

_____
_____
_____

Nutrition Center

Breakfast   Lunch

Dinner   Snacks

Drinks   Dessert

Water Log

1 2 3 4 5 6 7 8

Notes _____
_____
_____
_____
_____

Words to Live By *"Stop the habit of wishful thinking and start the habit of thoughtful wishes."*
—MARY MARTIN, AMERICAN ACTRESS

Today's Walk

How Far?_____

Strength Training? _____

How'd It Go? _____

Multivitamin ☐   Hours of Sleep ___

A Beautiful Thing

_____
_____
_____

Nutrition Center

Breakfast   Lunch

Dinner   Snacks

Drinks   Dessert

Water Log

1   2   3   4   5   6   7   8

Notes _____
_____
_____
_____
_____

Fab Food — Greens

- *Good source of folate, beta-carotene, flavonoids, vitamin C, and fiber*
- *Deeply colored leaves are more nutritious than lightly colored ones*
- *My favorite way to eat them: raw in salads*

Today's Walk

How Far?_____

Strength Training? _____

How'd It Go? _____

Multivitamin ☐   Hours of Sleep ___

A Beautiful Thing

_____
_____
_____

Nutrition Center

Breakfast   Lunch

Dinner   Snacks

Drinks   Dessert

Water Log

1 2 3 4 5 6 7 8

Notes _____
_____
_____
_____

Words to Live By *"Dedicate yourself to the good you deserve and desire for yourself. Give yourself peace of mind. You deserve to be happy. You deserve delight."*

—MARK VICTOR HANSEN, AMERICAN MOTIVATIONAL SPEAKER

Today's Walk

How Far?_____

Strength Training? _____

How'd It Go? _____

Multivitamin ☐   Hours of Sleep ____

A Beautiful Thing

_____
_____
_____

Nutrition Center	
Breakfast	Lunch
Dinner	Snacks
Drinks	Dessert

Water Log

① ② ③ ④ ⑤ ⑥ ⑦ ⑧

Notes _____
_____
_____

Reflections — *What do you think normal, healthy people should look like? At age thirty? At fifty? At seventy? Now think about your goals for your body. Are they realistic? Healthy? Do you hold yourself to a different standard than you do others?*

Today's Walk

How Far?_____

Strength Training? _____

How'd It Go? _____

Multivitamin ☐   Hours of Sleep ____

A Beautiful Thing

_____
_____
_____

Nutrition Center

Breakfast	Lunch
Dinner	Snacks
Drinks	Dessert

Water Log

[1] [2] [3] [4] [5] [6] [7] [8]

Notes _____
_____
_____
_____

Words to Live By *"Look at a day when you are supremely satisfied at the end. It's not a day when you lounge around doing nothing; it's when you've had everything to do, and you've done it."* —MARGARET THATCHER, BRITISH PRIME MINISTER

Today's Walk

How Far?_____

Strength Training? _____

How'd It Go?_____

Multivitamin ☐   Hours of Sleep ___

A Beautiful Thing

_____
_____
_____

Nutrition Center

Breakfast	Lunch
Dinner	Snacks
Drinks	Dessert

Water Log

1   2   3   4   5   6   7   8

Notes _____
_____
_____
_____

Fit Fact — *If you want to stay slim, it's best to start early. Two-thirds of overweight kids remain overweight as adults, and they are twice as likely to develop high blood pressure, heart disease, and diabetes.*

Today's Walk

How Far?_____

Strength Training? _____

How'd It Go?_____

Multivitamin ☐   Hours of Sleep ____

A Beautiful Thing

_____

_____

_____

Nutrition Center

Breakfast	Lunch
Dinner	Snacks
Drinks	Dessert

Water Log

1 2 3 4 5 6 7 8

Notes _____

_____

_____

_____

_____

Words to Live By "God gets you to the plate, but once you're there you're on your own."
—TED WILLIAMS, AMERICAN BASEBALL PLAYER

Today's Walk

How Far?_____

Strength Training? _____

How'd It Go?_____

Multivitamin ☐   Hours of Sleep ___

A Beautiful Thing

_____
_____
_____

Nutrition Center	
Breakfast	Lunch
Dinner	Snacks
Drinks	Dessert

Water Log

1 2 3 4 5 6 7 8

Notes _____
_____
_____
_____
_____

Fab Food — Almonds

- *Excellent source of vitamin E, potassium, iron, calcium, fiber, magnesium, and folate*
- *Good source of protein, healthy fats, and essential fatty acids*
- *Help prevent heart disease and stroke*
- *Use sparingly: substitute for unhealthy snack food*
- *My favorite way to eat them: as a midafternoon snack*

Today's Walk

How Far?_____

Strength Training? _____

How'd It Go? _____

Multivitamin ☐   Hours of Sleep ____

A Beautiful Thing

_____
_____
_____

Nutrition Center

Breakfast	Lunch
Dinner	Snacks
Drinks	Dessert

Water Log

🥛1 🥛2 🥛3 🥛4 🥛5 🥛6 🥛7 🥛8

Notes _____
_____

Words to Live By "As the family goes, so goes the
nation, and so goes the whole world in which we live."
—POPE JOHN PAUL II

Today's Walk

How Far?_____

Strength Training? _____

How'd It Go? _____

Multivitamin ☐   Hours of Sleep ___

A Beautiful Thing

_____
_____
_____

Nutrition Center

Breakfast	Lunch
Dinner	Snacks
Drinks	Dessert

Water Log

1 2 3 4 5 6 7 8

Notes _____
_____
_____
_____
_____

Reflections — Do you have any "toxic relationships" in your life–friends, coworkers, or family members who undercut your goals or self-esteem? Think about how your relationships with them developed, what each of you gets out of them, and how you might change the dynamic to one that is less harmful.

Today's Walk

How Far?_____

Strength Training? _____

How'd It Go? _____

Multivitamin ☐   Hours of Sleep ___

A Beautiful Thing

_____
_____
_____

Nutrition Center

Breakfast   Lunch

Dinner   Snacks

Drinks   Dessert

Water Log

Notes _____
_____
_____
_____

Monthly Check-In

Record below whichever numbers you've chosen to track, and compare with your original vital stats to see the improvement in your body in three months. Then use the space provided to take stock of all that you have achieved. Note what you still need to work on—along with the *actions* you will take in the next month to realize those goals.

Weight	_____	**Dress Size**	_____
Waist	_____	**Hips**	_____
Resting Heart Rate	_____	**Blood Pressure**	_____
Glucose	_____	**Total Cholesterol**	_____
LDL Cholesterol	_____	**Other**	_____

Goals met or exceeded

_____

_____

_____

_____

_____
_____
_____
_____
_____

Goals that still need attention, and actions you will take to meet them

_____
_____
_____
_____
_____
_____
_____
_____

New goals or dreams

_____
_____
_____
_____
_____
_____
_____
_____

Walking Wonder

Kim Hashim
FALLS CHURCH, VIRGINIA

Lost 129 pounds

I have been overweight since puberty and had been unable to lose any weight successfully. I decided in 2003 to have gastric-bypass surgery. As part of the approval process for my insurance company, I had to lose 5 percent of my weight in a six-month period. I had been walking outside, but I had severe plantar fasciitis. As a result of cortisone injections to control the pain and my walking on the uneven surfaces of the neighborhood, I tore the fascia in my foot and was in a cast for four weeks. After that, I decided to try Walk Away the Pounds. *I loved the energy and the ease of being able to do this program at home. I would get up early and do a mile in the morning before work and then do it again at night. I lost the weight needed to be approved for surgery. I had surgery in May 2004 and was very tired and weak for the first couple of months, but I continued to do one-mile walks.*

It was the perfect form of exercise for me at that time. It wasn't long before I began two-mile walks. Leslie is a great motivator and knows exactly when to encourage you to keep going! I recently did her three-mile tape for the first time, and I couldn't believe how far I had come in a year and a half. I have so much more energy. So far, I have lost 129 pounds!

The gastric bypass is a weight-loss tool, but it is not the magic bullet people think it is. At my support-group meetings, we talk about how easy it is to sabotage our weight loss, and how exercise is so important! I have told many people about the Walk Away the Pounds *program, how it is not dancing. We CAN do it! Even at 325 pounds, I could manage it. It is safe enough and powerful enough for people of all ages. My sixty-eight-year-old mother-in-law visited from Egypt, and I got her doing it with me. So I sent Leslie's one-mile tape back to Egypt with her, and my husband and I began doing the two-mile video. He has lost forty-five pounds! Yeah! Leslie is my friend and my helper in this journey, and she will continue to be the biggest part of my exercise program. I can't wait to see what the future brings.*

Words to Live By *"We are what we repeatedly do.
Excellence, then, is not an act, but a habit."*
—ARISTOTLE, GREEK PHILOSOPHER

Today's Walk

How Far?_____

Strength Training? _____

How'd It Go?_____

Multivitamin ☐   Hours of Sleep ___

A Beautiful Thing

_____
_____
_____

Nutrition Center

Breakfast	Lunch
Dinner	Snacks
Drinks	Dessert

Water Log

① ② ③ ④ ⑤ ⑥ ⑦ ⑧

Notes _____
_____
_____
_____
_____

Fit Fact — *During a two-mile walk, you burn your body weight in calories. If you weigh two hundred pounds, you burn two hundred calories on that walk.*

Today's Walk

How Far?_____

Strength Training? _____

How'd It Go?_____

Multivitamin ☐　　Hours of Sleep ___

A Beautiful Thing

_____
_____
_____

Nutrition Center

Breakfast	Lunch
Dinner	Snacks
Drinks	Dessert

Water Log

🥛1　🥛2　🥛3　🥛4　🥛5　🥛6　🥛7　🥛8

Notes _____
_____
_____
_____
_____

Words to Live By *"My life is one indivisible whole, and all my activities run into one another; and they all have their rise in my insatiable love for mankind."*

—MAHATMA GANDHI, INDIAN SPIRITUAL LEADER

Today's Walk

How Far?_____

Strength Training? _____

How'd It Go? _____

Multivitamin ☐   Hours of Sleep ____

A Beautiful Thing

_____

_____

_____

Nutrition Center

Breakfast	Lunch
Dinner	Snacks
Drinks	Dessert

Water Log

1   2   3   4   5   6   7   8

Notes _____

_____

_____

_____

Fab Food — Corn

- Good source of fiber, niacin, and potassium
- Contains carotenoids that help prevent eye disease
- Eat whole or stone-ground kernels for maximum benefit
- My favorite way to eat it: on the cob, of course!

Today's Walk

How Far?_____

Strength Training? _____

How'd It Go? _____

Multivitamin ☐   Hours of Sleep ____

A Beautiful Thing

_____

_____

_____

Nutrition Center

Breakfast   Lunch

Dinner   Snacks

Drinks   Dessert

Water Log

1   2   3   4   5   6   7   8

Notes _____

_____

_____

Words to Live By *"Life affords no higher pleasure that of surmounting difficulties, passing from one step of success to another, forming new wishes and seeing them gratified."* —SAMUEL JOHNSON, BRITISH AUTHOR

Today's Walk

How Far?_____

Strength Training? _____

How'd It Go?_____

Multivitamin ☐   Hours of Sleep ____

A Beautiful Thing

_____
_____
_____

Nutrition Center

Breakfast   Lunch

Dinner   Snacks

Drinks   Dessert

Water Log

① ② ③ ④ ⑤ ⑥ ⑦ ⑧

Notes _____
_____
_____
_____

Reflections — *What specific things do you want to do to celebrate once you've met your exercise/weight-loss goals? Think of as many as you can and write them down in today's Notes section.*

Today's Walk

How Far?_____

Strength Training? _____

How'd It Go? _____

Multivitamin ☐   Hours of Sleep ___

A Beautiful Thing

_____

_____

_____

Nutrition Center	
Breakfast	Lunch
Dinner	Snacks
Drinks	Dessert

Water Log

1   2   3   4   5   6   7   8

Notes _____

_____

_____

_____

_____

Words to Live By *"Everything you need you already have. You are complete right now, you are a whole, total person, not an apprentice person on the way to someplace else."* —WAYNE DYER, AMERICAN AUTHOR

Today's Walk

How Far?_____

Strength Training? _____

How'd It Go? _____

Multivitamin ☐   Hours of Sleep ___

A Beautiful Thing

_____
_____
_____

Nutrition Center	
Breakfast	Lunch
Dinner	Snacks
Drinks	Dessert

Water Log

🥛 🥛 🥛 🥛 🥛 🥛 🥛 🥛
1   2   3   4   5   6   7   8

Notes _____
_____
_____
_____

Fit Fact — *To burn fat, you need oxygen, so the process of burning fat happens best with exercises–such as walking!–that keep you breathing hard but not gasping.*

Today's Walk

How Far?_____

Strength Training? _____

How'd It Go? _____

Multivitamin ☐   Hours of Sleep ____

A Beautiful Thing

_____
_____
_____

Nutrition Center	
Breakfast	Lunch
Dinner	Snacks
Drinks	Dessert

Water Log

① ② ③ ④ ⑤ ⑥ ⑦ ⑧

Notes _____
_____
_____
_____
_____

Words to Live By *"Feeling sorry for yourself, and your present condition, is not only a waste of energy but the worst habit you could possibly have."*

—DALE CARNEGIE, AMERICAN MOTIVATIONAL SPEAKER

Today's Walk

How Far?_____

Strength Training? _____

How'd It Go? _____

Multivitamin ☐   Hours of Sleep ___

A Beautiful Thing

_____
_____
_____

Nutrition Center

Breakfast	Lunch
Dinner	Snacks
Drinks	Dessert

Water Log

🥛1 🥛2 🥛3 🥛4 🥛5 🥛6 🥛7 🥛8

Notes _____

_____
_____

Fab Food — Winter Squash

- *Excellent source of vitamin A*
- *Good source of vitamin C, potassium, fiber, and folate*
- *My favorite way to eat it: baked, with a roasted chicken for dinner*

Today's Walk

How Far?_____

Strength Training? _____

How'd It Go? _____

Multivitamin ☐   Hours of Sleep ____

A Beautiful Thing

_____
_____
_____

Nutrition Center	
Breakfast	Lunch
Dinner	Snacks
Drinks	Dessert

Water Log

1   2   3   4   5   6   7   8

Notes _____
_____
_____
_____

Words to Live By *"Tell me what you eat and I will tell you what you are."* —ANTHELME BRILLAT-SAVARIN, FRENCH GASTRONOME

Today's Walk

How Far?_____

Strength Training? _____

How'd It Go?_____

Multivitamin ☐   Hours of Sleep ___

A Beautiful Thing

_____
_____
_____

Nutrition Center

Breakfast	Lunch
Dinner	Snacks
Drinks	Dessert

Water Log

① ② ③ ④ ⑤ ⑥ ⑦ ⑧

Notes _____
_____
_____
_____
_____

Reflections — How much do TV and advertising influence what foods you choose to eat, what you drink, and what you think you should look like or act like? What changes could you make to gain more control over these decisions?

Today's Walk

How Far?_____

Strength Training? _____

How'd It Go? _____

Multivitamin ☐   Hours of Sleep ___

A Beautiful Thing

_____
_____
_____

Nutrition Center

Breakfast   Lunch

Dinner   Snacks

Drinks   Dessert

Water Log

Notes _____
_____
_____
_____
_____

Words to Live By "We first make our habits, and then our habits make us." —JOHN DRYDEN, BRITISH POET

Today's Walk

How Far?_____

Strength Training? _____

How'd It Go?_____

Multivitamin ☐　　　Hours of Sleep ___

A Beautiful Thing

_____
_____
_____

Nutrition Center

Breakfast　　　　　　　　Lunch

Dinner　　　　　　　　　Snacks

Drinks　　　　　　　　　Dessert

Water Log

1　2　3　4　5　6　7　8

Notes _____
_____
_____
_____
_____

Fit Fact — *Doing four hours per week of brisk exercise reduces your risk of breast cancer by 37 percent.*

Today's Walk

How Far?_____

Strength Training? _____

How'd It Go? _____

Multivitamin ☐   Hours of Sleep ____

A Beautiful Thing

_____
_____
_____

Nutrition Center

Breakfast   Lunch

Dinner   Snacks

Drinks   Dessert

Water Log

🥛1 🥛2 🥛3 🥛4 🥛5 🥛6 🥛7 🥛8

Notes _____
_____
_____
_____
_____

Words to Live By *"Faith makes all things possible; love makes all things easy."* —DWIGHT MOODY, AMERICAN EVANGELIST

Today's Walk

How Far?_____

Strength Training? _____

How'd It Go? _____

Multivitamin ☐   Hours of Sleep ___

A Beautiful Thing

_____
_____
_____

Nutrition Center

Breakfast	Lunch
Dinner	Snacks
Drinks	Dessert

Water Log

1 2 3 4 5 6 7 8

Notes _____
_____
_____
_____
_____

Fab Food — Strawberries

- *Excellent source of vitamin C*
- *Good source of fiber, flavonoids, potassium, and folate*
- *My favorite way to eat them: straight out of the bowl for dessert*

Today's Walk

How Far?_____

Strength Training? _____

How'd It Go? _____

Multivitamin ☐   Hours of Sleep ____

A Beautiful Thing

_____
_____
_____

Nutrition Center

Breakfast	Lunch
Dinner	Snacks
Drinks	Dessert

Water Log

1   2   3   4   5   6   7   8

Notes _____
_____
_____
_____

Words to Live By *"I believe God is managing affairs and that He doesn't need any advice from me. With God in charge, I believe everything will work out for the best in the end. So what is there to worry about?"*

—HENRY FORD, FOUNDER OF FORD MOTOR COMPANY

Today's Walk

How Far?_____

Strength Training? _____

How'd It Go? _____

Multivitamin ☐   Hours of Sleep ___

A Beautiful Thing

_____
_____
_____

Nutrition Center

Breakfast	Lunch
Dinner	Snacks
Drinks	Dessert

Water Log

1 2 3 4 5 6 7 8

Notes _____
_____

Reflections — *Do you spend a lot of time thinking about the past, or wishing you could change things that have happened? There are things we'd all like to change in our past–but none of us can! Focusing all our energy on the here and now is one of the best ways to stay effective and productive. Monitor your thinking and see how much time is spent worrying about past or future things beyond your control–then put all that energy into acting today!*

Today's Walk

How Far?_____

Strength Training? _____

How'd It Go? _____

Multivitamin ☐   Hours of Sleep ____

A Beautiful Thing

_____
_____
_____

Nutrition Center

Breakfast	Lunch
Dinner	Snacks
Drinks	Dessert

Water Log

1 2 3 4 5 6 7 8

Notes _____

Words to Live By *"Life takes on meaning when you become motivated, set goals and charge after them in an unstoppable manner."* —LES BROWN, AMERICAN MOTIVATIONAL SPEAKER

Today's Walk

How Far?_____

Strength Training? _____

How'd It Go? _____

Multivitamin ☐   Hours of Sleep ___

A Beautiful Thing

_____

_____

_____

Nutrition Center

Breakfast   Lunch

Dinner   Snacks

Drinks   Dessert

Water Log

🥛1 🥛2 🥛3 🥛4 🥛5 🥛6 🥛7 🥛8

Notes _____

_____

_____

_____

_____

Fit Fact — Women who exercise moderately during pregnancy have less back pain, more controlled weight gain, and easier deliveries than women who don't. They also have stronger immune systems, better circulation, and are less likely to deliver low-birth-weight babies.

Today's Walk

How Far?_____

Strength Training? _____

How'd It Go? _____

Multivitamin ☐   Hours of Sleep ____

A Beautiful Thing

_____
_____
_____

Nutrition Center

Breakfast	Lunch
Dinner	Snacks
Drinks	Dessert

Water Log

① ② ③ ④ ⑤ ⑥ ⑦ ⑧

Notes _____
_____
_____
_____

Words to Live By *"You can give without loving, but you cannot love without giving."*
—AMY CARMICHAEL, IRISH MISSIONARY

Today's Walk

How Far?_____

Strength Training? _____

How'd It Go? _____

Multivitamin ☐   Hours of Sleep ___

A Beautiful Thing

_____
_____
_____

Nutrition Center	
Breakfast	Lunch
Dinner	Snacks
Drinks	Dessert

Water Log

1 2 3 4 5 6 7 8

Notes _____
_____
_____
_____
_____

Fab Food — Wine

- Excellent source of flavonoids
- Markedly helps prevent heart disease and stroke
- Use sparingly: one glass per day
- My favorite way to drink it: a glass with dinner

Today's Walk

How Far?_____

Strength Training? _____

How'd It Go? _____

Multivitamin ☐   Hours of Sleep ____

A Beautiful Thing

_____
_____
_____

Nutrition Center	
Breakfast	Lunch
Dinner	Snacks
Drinks	Dessert

Water Log

1 2 3 4 5 6 7 8

Notes _____
_____
_____

Words to Live By *"Trust yourself. Create the kind of self that you will be happy to live with all your life. Make the most of yourself by fanning the tiny, inner sparks of possibility into flames of achievement."*

—FOSTER MCCLELLAN, AMERICAN AUTHOR

Today's Walk

How Far?_____

Strength Training? _____

How'd It Go? _____

Multivitamin ☐   Hours of Sleep ___

A Beautiful Thing

_____
_____
_____

Nutrition Center	
Breakfast	Lunch
Dinner	Snacks
Drinks	Dessert

Water Log

Notes _____
_____
_____

Reflections — *Sixteen weeks ago, I told you that the best indicator of fitness success is whether or not one keeps a journal. In what ways did this journal help you with your program? How would you modify it? Are there other aspects of your life in which a journal or day planner could be useful?*

Today's Walk

How Far?_____

Strength Training? _____

How'd It Go? _____

Multivitamin ☐   Hours of Sleep ____

A Beautiful Thing

_____
_____
_____

Nutrition Center	
Breakfast	Lunch
Dinner	Snacks
Drinks	Dessert

Water Log

Notes _____
_____
_____
_____

Walking Wonder

Diana DeTeresa

Staten Island, New York

Lost 110 pounds

Since October 2003, I have lost 110 pounds, and I owe my success to Weight Watchers and Leslie Sansone. I was an overweight person for as long as I can remember. I don't think I ever felt happy about myself. I dieted on and off, always gaining the weight back—and then some. I tried every diet imaginable. The common theme is that I never ever included exercise. I remember being weighed at the hospital after my first baby, and I weighed over three hundred pounds. I lost some weight, but I'd gained it all back by the time I became pregnant with my second daughter. My doctor warned me not to have another baby, because I was so unhealthy that I could have a stroke sitting in my car at a red light. The high blood pressure that had developed during my pregnancies was now here to stay. I was put on medication. My cholesterol was also high and I needed meds for that, as well. That should have scared me into changing my life, but it didn't. Eventually, my gallbladder was re-moved, and I was diagnosed with hypothyroidism. Again, I needed medication.

The summer I turned forty proved to be my turn-ing point. I came down with a bad case of bronchi-tis, which led to a diagnosis of bronchial asthma, acid-reflux disease, and sleep apnea—all obesity-related diseases. Medication alone would not fix me now. Finally, my mortality became an issue. I could not take a chance that my husband and two teenage daughters would have to face life without me. In October 2003, I walked into Weight Watchers, with a starting weight of 297. I have never been the same since. I knew I needed to incorporate exercise into my life, and I found Walk Away the Pounds *at a Best Buy. Leslie is so inspiring, and her laughter is conta-gious. She is like a part of the family! She has changed my life and my body. I am so self-assured, which is new. I am finally happy to be me, and that is an awesome accomplishment. It's me and a healthy lifestyle, which includes* Walk Away the Pounds—*forever.*

Four-Month Wrap-Up

THIS IS THE I DID IT! *PAGE.* If you've been filling the pages of this journal for four months, you've traveled far in your fitness journey. As with any trip, you're not quite the same person you were when you started. What a great time to stop and smell the roses of success. For you, those roses may include a whole new mental outlook.

Now is the time to go back to page 18 and fill in your "after" numbers to see just how far you've come. I'm sure you've been noting your physical improvements along the way—less body fat, more muscle, more energy—but answering the following questions will help you to become aware of all the other positive life changes that have been creeping up on you, and may help you to make any adjustments needed to your program as you begin the next four months. Keep having fun out there! I wish you all the success in the world!

1. How has your energy level changed after four months on your fitness program? What has that enabled you to do?

_____

_____

_____

_____

_____

_____

_____

_____

_____

2. What did you find most difficult about the program? What strategy did you use to overcome it? What advice would you give others just starting on the program?

_____

_____

_____

_____

_____

_____

_____

_____

_____

3. What was the most surprising improvement in your life resulting from your fitness program?

_____

_____

_____

_____

_____

_____

_____

_____

_____

4. Look back at the Dreamweaver pages, where you verbalized your dreams and goals. How many of them are coming true? How many do you need to keep working on? Are there some others that don't seem so important to you now? Any new goals come to you along the way?

_____

_____

_____

_____

_____

_____

_____

_____

_____

_____

5. As you prepare for your next four months, what changes will you make in your program? Will you walk farther or faster? Use heavier hand weights? Any additional diet changes you need to make?

_____

_____

_____

_____

_____

_____

_____

_____

_____

_____

_____

_____

6. How will you use your success in this program to further transform your life and the lives of those around you?

_____
_____
_____
_____
_____
_____
_____
_____
_____
_____

Also available wherever books are sold:

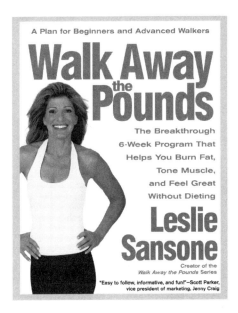

A Plan for Beginners and Advanced Walkers

Walk Away
the
Pounds

The Breakthrough
6-Week Program That
Helps You Burn Fat,
Tone Muscle,
and Feel Great
Without Dieting

Leslie
Sansone

Creator of the
Walk Away the Pounds Series

"Easy to follow, informative, and fun!"—Scott Parker,
vice president of marketing, Jenny Craig

If You Can Walk—
You Can *Walk Away the Pounds!*

"Leslie's energy, enthusiasm, and passion for walking are unparalleled—her program is simple and it really works!"
        —Jane Chesnutt, editor in chief, *Woman's Day*

CENTER
STREET

Where you live.

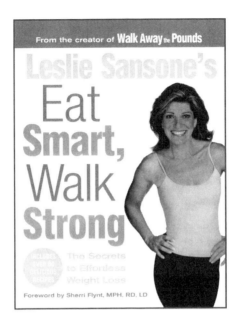